As I Lay Me Down To Die

When Suicide Is The Only Answer

by Toni Manofsin

©2016 USA

Intro:

Where does one begin when they reach the end? How do I tell my wife that I can't fight anymore? How do I tell her, after years of being an emasculated burden on her shoulders, that my last attempt to generate my own income to contribute has been detected by the sub-spirits and now the subhumans are even sabotaging that? I won't be making my own money to try to support my wife. Not now. To make money doing this, I had to promote my products. Promotion exposed what I was doing. It's so bad that all of my page reads and books sales came to a cartoonish screeching halt. If you're reading this, I probably died already and they no longer felt that they had to obscure it from your view. I was writing books as a last ditch effort, after all else has failed. It's embarrassing to exist like this, unable to support myself, relying on my wife as my provider. I think I've finally succumbed to the finality of it. I'm not getting out of this hole, not alive, anyway.

Chapter 1

Right now, I'm writhing this in extreme physical pain that more than rivals the emotional and psychological pain I've been enduring over the ongoing life-rape and emasculation carried out by the subhumans for their sub-spirit masters. The sub-spirits are partially artificial intelligence and have no empathy for anything living. If you are a threat to them, like I am, then you show up on their radar and they try to incapacitate you. And it can be really horrid if you're a dumb-ass, like I was, who doesn't even know that you're a targeted individual due to being perceived as a potential threat should you be awakened at some point.

I've pretty much reached the end of my rope. I have no hope of rescue nor intervention. Nobody is miraculously going to be concerned about my plight who might actually be able to help me. I can't find any good people to appeal to. It's as if I died and went into some sort of evil simulation of this simulation where everyone else is just an avatar who does the sub-spirits' bidding. So, those who would normally be inclined to reach out and help the less fortunate are instead being controlled to extreme omission. The animals suffer, unnecessarily. People like me suffer, for no reason other than for sport. I'm like entertainment for them now. No God or Devil rescues me from them. My pain entertains their feeble little minds and there are none left to defy it. My fate is to writhe in pain at their hands until I die.

The physical pain that I'm in is probably symptoms of Cancer. Although I am a burdensome wreck of a human to have for a spouse, my wife is still goddess enough to want to carry me through. She knows that this me that they turned me into is not the real me. I'm actually a very productive individual and this lack of lucrative productivity is tantamount to torture for me. So, my wife has been expressing concerns about the symptoms and she wants me to submit to a colonoscopy. She fears that the pain in my right shoulder, stemming from my neck and going across to and down my right arm is a sign that Cancer may have metastasized and gotten into my bones. I'm of the mindset that, if the Cancer has traveled that far, then it's already too late. That's a long way from my colon for the Cancer to have traveled for me to still have a chance at survival. I'm a dead man, anyway; the walking dead, just waiting to happen.

Chapter 2

I held out this long out of spite and due to faith. Those two forces kept me holding on while I continued to work my ass off in a vain attempt to break the chains of poverty that kept me so solidly rooted to Loserville. I had faith that God was not a liar and that I would eventually reap a harvest for all of the good seeds I sowed into various things, like into the music industry. I held on, thinking that God would miraculously force a harvest for me out of this shithole and I could spite them with the enormous victory it would be. They would no longer be able to gloat about being stronger than both God and Lucifer as they robbed me of what I was long overdue. I wanted them to have to eat their words and to have to admit that God DOES provide, that He was NOT a liar, and that people DO reap what they sow. Even now, they laugh and say "Good luck with that."

I wanted revenge. If I wanted bloody revenge, I would have resorted to it. I come from a violent background and getting that kind of revenge is easy for me. I can burn down an enemy's home with him sleeping inside without the slightest tinge of remorse. I can invest thirty seconds of my time under the car of an enemy and cause it to explode when he turns on the ignition and, again, I'd feel no remorse. If someone fucks with me, I can easily kill them and everyone who tries to protect them from me and not feel the slightest bit of regret about it. So, if I wanted that kind of revenge, I could of already gotten it. Then, I could have taken their money and possessions and I wouldn't be in this position, financially, that I'm in right now.

I wanted POSITIVE revenge. The kind of revenge that would have had me being all kinds of successful and prosperous beyond the wildest dreams of my enemies, to make them green with envy and full of regret that they can't partake in my booty. I wanted God to stomp the dog-fuck out of them like that. It probably made me look like a gold-digger to those who can't understand what it's like to always be the underdog who never gets a leg up.

I've never had a victory, ever. I've never had a significant other, male nor female, who would not betray me if the right opportunity presented itself. I'm a swinger so, if my spouse wants to fuck someone, I'm not going to cock-block. Hell, I might even try to set it up. So the infidelity is always something beyond just physical desire. It's a desire to fuck me over, to rape me with secrets being kept from me for another human with every passing second that those secrets are kept from me for that other person. It puts me on the outside, not as close as the one who has secrets with someone who is supposed to be connected to me on a stronger level.

I would have settled for the faithful significant other. That would have been more valuable to me than all of the revenge that the success and wealth would have brought. Understand that I don't mean chaste when I refer to faithfulness and fidelity. I'd expect a heads up if she or he is fucking someone else, though. But I'm so oversexed, perverted, and such a chameleon that I don't see how anyone could need something more.

I'm willing to do whatever my partner desires, even when it involves other entities. I'm the ultimate partner, in that respect; if you want someone who you can share your perversions and kinks with instead of hiding them all the time. But I'm being deprived of even having that one person that I can be connected to like that...It's an even bigger jab when you consider that I was not race nor gender specific in my desire for this entity. It's like seven billion rejections, all at once.

Chapter 3

You know, my teeth come out and I love to perform oral. I'm sexy and smart. I shape-shift from masculine to feminine effortlessly. I'm well-hung. I'm not a drunk nor a chemical toilet. Lately I've been having to eat a lot of Tylenol 3 with Codeine due to the pain being too much for the Marijuana to relieve on its own. But I don't drink or do drugs, for the most part.

    I smoke a lot of Marijuana and drink coffee and smoke some cigarettes. On occasion, I may smoke a little Crack with someone to get "suck happy" (during the come-down) for a sexual encounter where I will be performing as the female entity doing a lot of receiving of big cock. That's about it, though. I don't like any of the other stuff. Maybe some acid or mescaline, once in awhile. But it's been years since I've indulged in anything other than pot, and Tylenol, really.

For years I had a feminine plump shapely butt. It's as if I was physically already part female. Even my legs were feminine. My hands are on the small side, too. And my feet are small and pretty. But lately, I've been losing a lot of weight. I went down more than twenty pounds to 156 pounds, rapidly, like within 6 months time. I'm shorter, 5' 9 or 10" or thereabouts; so the lower weight works for everything except for my face and my butt. With less fat on my face, I look older and more masculine. With less fat on my butt, I'm losing that pretty feminine roundness I managed to retain all of these years. With less fat on my legs, they look more manly, too. I was already battling gruesome scars on my left leg from a freak accident (I was hit by my own car) that resulted in me briefly dying on an operating table. Getting older, with no help from female hormones, is starting to take a toll: It's making me less passable, and I was already not passable, as it was.

So the whole world seems complicit in the deprivation campaign that hinders me from succeeding and prospering at something (anything, anything at all, sucking cock, taking it up my ass, anything, I don't care). That deprivation of success and prosperity stops me dead in my tracks to fulfill my agendas which all require funding: Building and operating animal sanctuaries and homeless shelters requires money. Buying a ranch to move my wife and our family of rescue animals to costs money. Retaining a competent attorney who can get my driver's license restored requires money. The surgeries, procedures, and hormones I need for transforming my body to my proper gender all cost money.

They have me on an endless quest to get money to do the good things that other humans should be actively trying to fund and support. It's like the sub-spirits want me to worship money, which goes against my religious beliefs, so they control the world to ignore my plight and my super cool lucrative venture opportunities...I don't like thinking about money or new ways to try to earn it, nor trying to beg for it. I just want to market a skill that I enjoy doing and make my money the hard, old-fashioned way, that's all. I never wanted special treatment nor a handout. I always had faith that I would succeed if I were helped to do so and then I could simply reciprocate the blessing and it would be paid back...

It was never my intention to become a beggar who asks for donations on all of my websites. I was never very effective at it, never being able to motivate a chain of donations or a rally of support for any of the causes that I've represented over the years.

Chapter 4

So I'm getting uglier and more masculine as I age due to a lack of funding for the basic hormones I should be on to reverse this process that my body is going through. I was hoping to become a secret sex slave to a billionaire who would hide me away and pay for my transformations and give me an allowance to pursue my philanthropic agendas.

I'd hoped to get hidden away on a huge ranch that was in my wife's name, with her hired as one of my personal assistants, so that I could live out my trans-formative year as a woman (required by law for GRS) in private. I wanted my billionaire master to buy me a variety of state of the art sex toys, mechanical and stationary; after springing for the more complicated vaginal surgeries that require using a portion of my colon to make my vagina deeper and able to self-lubricate. My dreams had me becoming the most awesome female fuck toy that man's money and science could create out of me...

But the donor never materialized. Even billionaires were mind-controlled against me, when I was an object that many of them should have wanted to collect. I'm the prime sample that every perv should want, someone who fucks like a child who just got turned on to early orgasms, who also possesses an adolescent innocence. My greatest personality traits are the ability to keep secrets and loyalty to those I become obligated to. So any rich perv who has a fetish for fucking kids or someone with an innocent mind should have been all over me.

Then, there was the option to participate in what I will turn into, to help make decisions about what I will transform into: How many billionaires were robbing themselves of that power over me that would've given them so much satisfaction far beyond the sex that they would also get? See what I mean? If you're targeted, even billionaires will rob themselves of rare one of a kind collectibles just to keep you deprived. Even if I'm exactly what so many of them secretly desire.

I despise the thought that, as another second passes, they are getting more victories over me. With every passing second, they are defeating the spiritual laws of sowing and reaping that God and Lucifer agreed would be the controlling forces at play here. They get to deprive me of driving and earning an income doing what I love to do, which has a domino effect on everything else that is negatively effected by the lack of money.

They seem to be able to throw sand in my wells no matter where I dig them. They really do appear to have God and Lucifer defeated. I was a representative to both parties, so that means that I am defeated, as well. If Lucifer were in power, they wouldn't be able to control humans to neglect and abuse his animals or to molest children or to treat women like second class citizens or to beat down the taxpayer heroes. Lucifer doesn't condone any of that shit. Lucifer also wouldn't tolerate them desecrating his craft of music while cock-blocking real musicians of my caliber, either. So not even Lucifer can help me now.

Every day I wake up here I'm at a loss. I don't know how I'm supposed to get out of this pit. I've been stuck here for so long that I've become convinced that it can't be done, I'll never get out. This is how I die; alone, lonely, deprived of all things that I desired, sad, ill, in pain, and angry. I've worked harder than most only to have far less than most. I never should've tried. I could've been like my brothers and just lived a life of getting fucked up every day, with no concern for anything else.

Hell, my one brother is such a drunken chemical toilet that he can't even be imposed upon to get up off of his ass to let the dog go potty outside. Yet that drunken piece of shit is more loved by my family and regarded as more valuable and worthy of love than I am. If I were exactly the same way as him, they would adopt a double standard that vilifies me for being the same way as him while glorifying him for being the way that they rebuke me for being. It's so ridiculous. I came from a family who eats their own...Unless you're a drunken pedophilic piece of shit (in which case, then they're enablers).

Chapter 5

Yeah, I don't know how I can be expected to carry on like this. I'm writhing in pain, constantly. I have no musical equipment, not even an old acoustic 6-string to play on. I have no family. I have no friends. I have a house full of furry family depending on me to provide and the vultures are coming to take my ability to even do that away from me. How can I continue to live and allow the subhumans to have the victory of taking quality of life from my little animals?

If I die, maybe people will sympathize with my wife and help her, which will help the animals relying on me to outsmart the sub-spirits and the subhumans under their control to deprive me and starve me out.

I feel so sorry for my animals, how they're under fire just for being mine. I cry as I pet them, knowing that my time with them is coming to an end. I even had nightmares that my wife died and I was unable to support us and I had to betray them by taking them to a shelter because I became homeless...

That dream is too easy to make come true since they empowered terrorists to pose as government to enable the Secretary of State to illegally deprive me of my driver's license for my entire adult life over a few childhood driving under the influence of alcohol offenses. I haven't had a driver's license for 34 years, since I was 18 years old. I fought to get it back, multiple times, only to find that they are never going to let it happen. I'm being life-raped by the terrorists with every passing second that I'm illegally deprived of my driver's license. I want to defeat them badly enough to die to make it happen. It may be a final victory for them: They'll think they won, that they drove me from the planet without with slightest victory nor hint of success. But it deprives them of doing it to me for more passing seconds, which is a victory, in and of itself.

So I've come to this strange place where the only answer, the only viable solution, is for me to die. I have no other options. I'm all tapped out for amazing ideas that would work for others but always fail for me. They deprive my wife to deprive me, which is negatively effecting her health. She needs extra money for smart liposuction to defy the Lipedema that she's been stricken with as unwitting science experiment to a crazed tyrannical regime of fucktards. She's blown up to 300 pounds. She's not lazy, nor is she gluttonous. She's a targeted individual, too; but in a different category. They passively targeted her demographic. And she only comes under direct targeting radar now in order to keep me down.

They don't want to let me get out of this hole because I may get my sex change and then make a bunch of best case scenario prophecies involving Lucifer and my sexual energy force come true. Then, they lose the power to cause unnecessary suffering and God and Lucifer can reclaim this simulation mechanism...But that's the subject of other books, not this one.

In Closing:

So I'm a defeated entity who has but one option to escape this fate worse than death. I defied it for years. My reasons were varied: Spite. Revenge. Hatred. And probably cowardice.

I think that I was probably too afraid to kill myself before. There was also always this thought that would stop me: "You're gonna' kill yourself today and your miracle was going to manifest tomorrow and you won't be here to receive it, giving them an even greater victory." I would then hold on out of spite again, not wanting to give them that level of victory, that I would kill myself the day before my liberation was to manifest. It's been a constant battle like that. I want out of this bad enough to die to make it happen. By getting it without dying, I'd hoped to rub their faces in it. But it's getting pretty bad and I think I may be wise to just cut my losses and bail. I'm not accomplishing anything with this unwarranted procrastination. I look like a coward who's too afraid to do what's necessary.

It appears as though my mental illness has finally caught up with me. But maybe it's the other way around. Maybe my mental illness was in the delusion that I would one day escape the parameters of this existence while still alive. Maybe it's evidence of being cured of my mental illness to finally have the clarity to understand that dying is my only way out of this constant suffering. There's no God coming to rescue me; not now, not tomorrow, not ever. To stay alive is like letting them dupe me into giving them how many more seconds of victory? I'm not willing to let them have that anymore. It's time for me to put a stop to this. It's not going to get better. I'm a coward to allow it to continue.

The End

This book is not meant to encourage nor condone suicide. The writer has endured a long life of failure to reach the conclusions made here. If you are considering committing suicide, please seek help immediately. Your situation is nowhere near as bad as what was endured before coming to this end. Seek counseling before making your final decision.

www.ingramcontent.com/pod-product-compliance
Lightning Source LLC
Chambersburg PA
CBHW070720210526
45170CB00021B/1389